I believe this book is an excellent idea. It is simply written, easy to understand, accurate and concise. In these times of sexual fear, it can serve as a valuable educational source for all who are sexually active.

Ken Peters, M.D., Director
South Drive Medical Clinic
Mountain View, CA

*Play Safe* is styled in a way that provides easy access to a number of different questions, such as: What will lower my risk of getting STDs? Is there a vaccine to prevent STDs? Do birth control pills prevent STDs? What are the advantages of using a condom? These are just a few of the issues which the authors address in a neat and concise manner. *Play Safe* does not concern itself with disease-causing organisms, but with how to understand and avoid getting STDs.

There are many books on the market that have good information about sexually transmitted diseases. Now there is a book that finally addresses the type of questions frequently asked by the average person needing information about STDs.

I would highly recommend *Play Safe* to anyone who has an interest in this modern-day health problem.

Remy Lazarowicz, Director
VD National Hotline

# PLAY SAFE

## How to Avoid Getting Sexually Transmitted Diseases

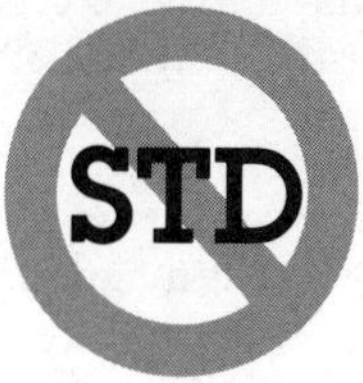


Bea Mandel and Byron Mandel

Preface by Mary-Ann Shafer, M.D.



Center for Health Information
P.O. Box 4636 Foster City, CA 94404

This book is intended for educational purposes and should not be used as a guide for the diagnosis of and/or treatment of any disease. The reader needing guidance on any particular health care problem should seek the help of a licensed health professional of his or her choice.

Discounts can be made available on purchase of multiple copies. Contact: Center for Health Information
P.O. Box 4636
Foster City, CA 94404
(415) 345-6669

ISBN: 0-932567-00-2 Softcover
Library of Congress Catalog Card Number 85-070063
Printed in the United States of America

# CONTENTS

# PREFACE

For the first time, there is a book in print that addresses "all the things you ever wanted to know about sexually transmitted diseases but were afraid to ask." *Play Safe* is a unique and valuable resource for anyone who is sexually active or desires to know more about sexually transmitted diseases (STDs). The authors have carefully researched the subject of sexually transmitted diseases and have wisely chosen an effective question-and-answer format to present critical information regarding STD prevention and treatment. *Play Safe* provides accurate, easy-to-understand information that can be effectively used by teenagers, college students, adults, teachers, counselors, health professionals, and parents.

As a clinician working with young adults, I am often approached by teenagers asking questions about sexually transmitted diseases. *Play Safe* can provide these young people with the information they seek. It is particularly important that young people receive this information, since sexually active teenagers, especially girls, are at the greatest risk of becoming infected by STDs. In the past, much attention has been directed toward preventing pregnancy in teenage girls, and relatively little attention has been paid to the major cause of infertility in young women—pelvic infections caused by STDs. Similarly, teenage boys often do not receive critical information about STDs until it is too late. *Play Safe* brings home the important message that disease prevention is the key to teenage health care.

Adults of all ages can profit from reading *Play Safe.* Designed to be used as a "self-help" educational tool, this book can help young and old alike to decrease their chances of getting an STD and, in the process, establish a safer and healthier lifestyle. *Play Safe* addresses common concerns of both single people and couples, regardless of sexual attitudes or lifestyle. Health considerations of pregnant women are also discussed.

Teachers and counselors who work with young adults will also find *Play Safe* to be a valuable reference source and teaching aid. Professionals will be pleased to find information about STDs (some of which is sensitive in nature) presented simply, clearly, and directly. *Play Safe* is an excellent resource for public school and college libraries, as well as in the home.

With growing public awareness of STDs, particularly through recent media coverage, it is important that all doctors, nurses, and other health care providers be well informed about the prevention and treatment of STDs. Because STDs affect people of all ages, ethnic backgrounds, and economic situations, all health care professionals should be aware of patient concerns, and be prepared to answer questions about STDs as they come up. Again, *Play Safe* provides a welcome and effective resource for health care professionals working in a clinic setting or in private practice.

Finally, I would like to note two features of *Play Safe* that I think readers will find especially useful. One, "Where to Get More Help," provides a comprehensive listing of STD resources, advising the reader where to go for additional help and information about STDs. The other feature, "Definitions of Terms and Diseases," provides an excellent overview of commonly used terminology associated with STDs.

I would like to take this opportunity to commend the authors of *Play Safe* for providing a much needed, simply written informational guide to understanding the prevention and treatment of sexually transmitted diseases. As the authors themselves say, the only way to control the spread of STDs is to better understand them, ourselves, and our partners. This book is a wonderful step towards increased understanding and, hopefully, towards the control of STDs and their consequences.

Mary-Ann Shafer, M.D.
Assistant Professor of Pediatrics
Associate Director, Division of
Adolescent Medicine
Director of Adolescent Clinics
University of California, San Francisco

# INTRODUCTION

**Do you know that . . .**

- Sexually transmitted diseases (STDs) are extremely contagious.
- There are more than 20 different diseases that can be sexually transmitted.
- The risk of getting an STD is greater than ever—over 10 million people in the United States get some form of STD each year.
- Some STDs can lead to serious medical complications—even death—if not properly treated.
- You can have an STD and have no noticeable symptoms.
- The more sexual partners you have, the more likely you are to get an STD.
- You can spread an STD to other people and not know it.
- Precautions can be taken that will reduce your risk of getting an STD.
- The more you know about STDs, the less likely you are to get one.

If some of these facts come as news to you, you are not alone. Most people know very little about sexually transmitted diseases (STDs). In fact, lack of knowledge is one of the main reasons that more and more people are getting STDs each year in this country. Most people do not recognize the risks involved in sexual contact, nor do they know what can be done to reduce these risks.

The purpose of *Play Safe* is to provide you with important information about the prevention of STDs, and to tell you what to do if you should get one. This book explains:

- How to identify common situations that can lead to getting an STD
- What you can do to reduce your risk of getting an STD
- How to recognize STD symptoms
- What to do if you or your partner gets an STD
- How to help other people understand what they can do to prevent the spread of STDs

Throughout this book, we have tried to provide answers to the most commonly asked questions about STDs. You will probably find that some of the information presented here clears up some doubts or confusion you might have about STDs. Other information may not seem particularly useful to you right now, but may become useful at some time in the future. The knowledge you gain by reading this book may someday help you or a friend to better deal with an STD problem.

We have specifically avoided making moral or philosophical judgments about anyone's sexual practices. What we have tried to do is impress upon you, the reader, the importance of being well informed about STDs. As long as you are sexually active (even if it is with only one long-term partner), you risk becoming infected by an STD. It is up to you to understand what this risk means, and to take the necessary precautions.

*Play Safe* does not attempt to answer technical questions about the diagnosis or treatment of STDs, nor does it discuss very much anatomy, biology, or physiology. These subjects are covered in a variety of other books that can be found in a bookstore or in your local library. A health professional is probably your best overall source of information, and can usually answer any specific questions you may have about the prevention, symptoms, and treatment of STDs.

Once you have read *Play Safe*, let other people know that you have information about a very important subject. And let them know that you are interested in sharing this knowledge. It is only by communicating with others about STDs that we can hope to control the spread of infection.

# CHAPTER ONE

# KNOW THEIR NAMES AND THE RISKS

## What are STDs and how do people get them?

Sexually transmitted diseases (STDs) are a group of diseases that are passed on from one person to another by intimate physical contact (sexual relations, other close body contact, and occasionally kissing).

The term STD is used to refer to all sexually transmitted diseases, although not all STDs involve sexual contact, and some do not affect the sexual organs. STDs are commonly referred to as venereal disease or VD, meaning related to sexual relations.

**What are the most common STDs?**

Until recently, gonorrhea and syphilis were the most common STDs. Now, herpes, venereal warts, chlamydia, and various forms of vaginitis are becoming equally common.

## How many STDs are there?

In all, more than 20 different diseases are now considered to be sexually transmitted.

In addition to the more common STDs mentioned previously, less common STDs include: lymphogranuloma venereum (LGV), chancroid, hepatitis B, and certain intestinal diseases.

Several parasitic diseases, such as crabs and scabies, are also classified as STDs since they are easily spread from person to person through physical contact.

The *Definitions of Terms and Diseases* in the back of this book provides a brief explanation of sexually transmitted diseases.

**What are the most serious STDs?**

Acquired Immunodeficiency Syndrome (AIDS) is a life-threatening disease for which there is no effective treatment. Syphilis is also a very serious STD that can be fatal, but only if it is not successfully treated.

Gonorrhea and chlamydia are potentially serious diseases if not properly treated. Both can result in pelvic inflammatory disease (PID), which can lead to permanent sterility in men and women, or ectopic pregnancy.

Some studies have associated herpes and venereal warts with cervical cancer in women.

**How serious is herpes?**

In general, herpes is not a seriously disabling or life-threatening disease, however periodic flare-ups can cause physical and emotional distress.

A person who has herpes is often angry or resentful towards the partner who gave it to him or her. Also, the fear of accidentally passing along the virus to another partner may cause the infected person to avoid sexual activity altogether. In addition, people who do not have herpes are often afraid of getting it from a partner who may be infected, even if he or she has no symptoms.

It is estimated that 20 million people have herpes in the United States today.

## What is AIDS and how is it spread?

The recently identified disease called Acquired Immunodeficiency Syndrome (AIDS) appears to be caused by a virus referred to as the Human Type Leukemia Virus III (HTLV III). So far the disease is not well understood, and there is no effective treatment for it.

AIDS causes a breakdown of the immune system, making it impossible to fight off infections. Even illnesses such as colds and flu become life-threatening to the person who has AIDS; victims usually die within three years after being diagnosed.

Investigators have identified several groups as having the greatest risk of getting AIDS:

- Homosexual men who have intimate contact with many partners
- People who inject drugs into their veins
- Haitians
- Hemophiliacs and other blood recipients (these people require blood transfusions that could be contaminated with the AIDS virus)

While heterosexuals are not, at this time, at high risk for AIDS, there have been a number of recently reported cases of heterosexual men and women who have gotten the disease.

AIDS does not appear to be spread through casual (non-sexual) contact with an infected person.

# CHAPTER TWO

# HOW STDs ARE TRANSMITTED (AND HOW THEY ARE NOT)

## Why are so many people getting sexually transmitted diseases?

In the past, many people had only one sexual partner throughout their lifetime. Now, it is quite common for people to have numerous sexual partners. Unfortunately, increasing one's sexual contacts also increases the risk of getting a sexually transmitted disease.

Adding to the problem is the fact that people who pass on STDs to their partners often do not realize that they are contagious. For example, Tom spends the night with Jane. Tom later finds out that he has an STD, and thinks that he got it from Jane. Actually, he got it from Linda a few days before he spent the night with Jane. If Jane and Linda have no noticeable symptoms, and if Tom does not tell either woman about his condition, both women may spread the disease to other people.

The more sexual partners one has, the greater the chance of getting an STD from someone who may not realize that he or she is infected. Often, the contagious person is someone just like you— someone who is responsible and caring, and who would never knowingly pass on a disease to another person.

## How are STDs spread from person to person?

To get an STD infection, you must have close contact with someone who is already infected.

There are various ways that disease can be spread. For example, if someone has a genital infection (involving the sex organs), contact with that person's genitals will increase your risk of getting the infection. If an infection is in or around the mouth, contact with the infected person's mouth may transmit the disease. Some diseases can be spread by contact between one person's genitals and another person's mouth. If there is any contact with the rectal area, infection can also be spread to or from that part of the body.

Crabs, which are actually tiny insects, are commonly transmitted by sexual or intimate contact, but may also be passed on by close body contact or by wearing the clothes of an infected person. You can also get crabs by using the towel, sheets, or sleeping bag of someone who is infected.

**What are my chances of getting an STD?**

If you have sexual contact with someone who has an infection, the risk of getting that infection is extremely high. Infections are also occasionally transmitted by kissing. Your ability to resist STDs may vary, depending on your overall state of health, and how easy it is for you to resist diseases in general.

Again, the more people with whom you have intimate contact, the greater your risk of becoming infected.

**Is it possible to have an STD if I have not had recent sexual contact and have no symptoms?**

Yes. Many infections do not cause immediate symptoms.

Some infections become obvious within one or two days; others may not produce symptoms for several months, or even a year or longer. Venereal warts, for example, may be present for several weeks or months before producing any noticeable symptoms. (Women may have warts on their cervix that can only be detected with a pelvic examination.) If you have been exposed to an STD but have no symptoms, it is still possible that you have been infected.

**What parts of my body are most likely to be infected by STDs?**

The most commonly infected parts of the body are the warm, moist areas around the sex organs—the vagina in women, and the penis and opening of the penis in men.

The rectum, mouth, and throat also can be easily infected. Other areas that may become infected are the eyes and any open sores on the skin that come in direct contact with an infection.

## Can STDs spread from one part of my body to another?

Yes. If you touch an infected sore or blister, and then touch another part of your body, the infection can be spread.

While the skin serves as a barrier against infection, mucous membranes such as the moist areas of the eyes, nose, mouth, and genitals do not. Also, cuts or sores on the skin provide entry points for infectious organisms.

If you have sores or blisters on your body, take extra care to wash your hands with soap and water after touching them. To help prevent the spread of infection, it is a good idea to avoid sharing washcloths and towels with other people.

Just as STDs can be spread from one part of your body to another, they can also be spread to another person's body. You can infect another person by touching your sore and then touching someone else without first washing your hands. Similarly, you can become infected by touching another person's sore and then touching yourself.

Close physical contact with someone who has sores anywhere on his or her body can be risky. Even if you intend to be cautious, your good intentions may be forgotten during sexual excitement.

## Can one STD become another?

No, one disease cannot become another. Gonorrhea cannot become syphilis. Herpes cannot become gonorrhea.

Every sexually transmitted disease is different—each has different causes, each is diagnosed with different tests, and each is treated with special medication for a specific length of time.

**If I have had one kind of STD, can I get another?**

Yes. Just because you have had one disease does not mean you cannot get another. Also, if you have an STD that has been cured, you can get the same disease again if you have contact with an infected person.

It is also possible to have more than one disease at a time. For example, you can have both gonorrhea and syphilis, herpes and vaginitis, or any of a number of other disease combinations.

**Can STDs be transmitted through saliva?**

Yes, saliva can carry organisms that cause disease. For example, the virus for oral herpes is present in saliva; the hepatitis B virus is also carried in bodily fluids.

**Can I get STDs by sharing a hypodermic needle to inject drugs?**

Yes. Some of the most serious STDs, such as hepatitis B and AIDS, are transmitted through the blood system. Drug users who share needles with other people increase their risk of getting a serious or fatal STD.

**Are canker sores or cold sores a form of STD?**

Canker sores are not considered to be a form of STD; cold sores are a common form of herpes, but are not usually sexually transmitted.

Canker sores are generally caused by excess acidity in the mouth or a change in the bacteria that normally live in the mouth. These sores are sometimes mistaken for herpes (and vice versa), and may be confused with the hard chancre that is the first symptom of syphilis.

Caused by the herpes simplex virus, cold sores are quite contagious. People with cold sores on their mouths should avoid kissing or being kissed by others until the sores have healed and disappeared.

If you have a sore that you think may be related to an STD, it is best to have it looked at by a health professional.

**Can bisexual or gay men get STDs?**

Yes. Common STDs seen in bisexual and/or gay men include syphilis, gonorrhea, chancroid, chlamydia, herpes, venereal warts, and a variety of intestinal parasites. Homosexual men are at greater risk of getting AIDS than is the general population, but the reason for this is not yet clear.

**Can lesbians or bisexual women get STDs?**

Yes. Like anyone else, lesbians and bisexual women can get STDs through sexual contact with an infected partner.

The rate of infection among lesbians, however, is generally lower than that of heterosexual women. The most common infections among lesbians are yeast infections, herpes, and nonspecific vaginitis. Because of differences in the sexual practices of homosexual men and women, lesbians are less likely to get the kinds of diseases that are common among gay men.

**Can unborn babies get STDs?**

Yes. Because a mother and her unborn baby share the same blood, infections that are carried in the blood, such as syphilis and cytomegalovirus, can be passed on from mother to child.

Some of these infections can cause severe damage to an unborn baby if the mother fails to get medical treatment. Other diseases, like herpes, do not affect the unborn baby, but can get passed on during the birth process as the baby travels through the mother's birth canal.

**Can newborn babies be affected by STDs?**

If the mother of a newborn baby has an infection at the time of delivery, the infection can be passed on to the baby as it goes through the birth canal.

Both gonorrhea and chlamydia organisms can be spread during the birth process, causing blindness in newborn infants. (Most hospitals now use eyedrops or ointments in newborns to prevent the possibility of this occurring.) Untreated chlamydia can cause pneumonia in newborns, and herpes can cause a systemic (throughout the body) viral infection, resulting in severe kidney, spleen, and brain damage.

Because the immune system of newborn babies is not fully developed during the first several months of life, even the simplest infections are difficult for newborns to resist. For this reason, it is important that friends or relatives with cold sores (herpes) be particularly careful around newborns so that their virus is not passed on to the baby.

**Can children get STDs?**

Yes. Crabs, scabies, and herpes are commonly passed on to children through nonsexual contact.

If a child is diagnosed as having a disease usually transmitted only through sexual contact, sexual abuse should be suspected, and the case should be further investigated by the family physician or other health professional.

**Can anyone get an STD?**

Yes. STDs can affect rich or poor, young or old, black, white, brown, or yellow. A person need only be exposed to the virus, bacteria, or other disease agent—the organism will do the rest.

## Can I get STDs from masturbating?

STDs are transmitted through direct contact with an infected person. If you touch an infected area of another person's body with your hand, and then use the same hand to masturbate, there is some chance of getting infected yourself.

Open sores on a person's hands are the most likely source of such infections. Check your own hands, and the hands of people with whom you are intimate. Look for sores, warts, or other blemishes that may spread infection.

**Can I get STDs from a prostitute?**

Yes. Prostitutes can spread STD infections.

Since numerous sexual partners increase one's chances of becoming infected, prostitutes, in general, are more likely to get STDs. Prostitutes who have many partners are also more likely to spread disease, particularly if they do not have periodic medical check-ups.

**Can I get an STD at a party?**

Yes, but only if you have intimate contact with an infected person.

If you go to a party and have sexual contact with someone you've just met, obviously your risk of getting an infection is increased. In other words, it is what you do, not where you do it, that determines your risk of infection.

Whenever possible, it is helpful to exchange names, addresses, and telephone numbers with your sexual partners, regardless of where you meet them, so that you can notify each other should either of you discover that you have an STD.

## Can I get STDs from toilet seats?

Generally speaking, you cannot get infected from an inanimate object such as a toilet seat.

Most organisms that transmit sexual diseases need the human body to survive and multiply. Specifically, these organisms require the warmth and moisture found in mucous membranes such as the tissue inside the mouth, vagina, and urinary tract. A toilet seat, for the most part, does not provide this type of environment.

Crabs and scabies, because they are insects, can survive for long periods of time outside the human body. However, one would have to perch in quite a strange position in order to have one's genitals infected by organisms that might be present on a toilet seat.

**Can I get STDs from sitting in a hot tub or bathtub?**

Heat, detergent, and other chemicals kill most disease-causing organisms that may be present in tubs. However, if you have sexual contact with someone in a hot tub or bathtub, you still risk becoming infected.

**Can I get an STD from using someone else's towel?**

For the most part, STDs are transmitted from person to person. Disease-causing organisms generally cannot survive long enough on articles such as towels and washcloths to infect another person. Crabs, scabies, and other small parasites, however, can be spread in this way. For this reason, it makes sense to avoid using another person's towel or other personal items whenever possible.

## Am I more likely to get STDs in a large city?

Government statistics show that the highest percentage of STD cases occurs in the largest cities.

Because larger populations provide greater opportunities for contact and, therefore, a higher rate of infection, new diseases often are first identified in large cities and then gradually spread throughout the rest of the country.

# CHAPTER THREE

# PREVENTION IS THE NAME OF THE GAME

### What will increase my risk of getting an STD?

The less you know about your sexual partner, the more likely you are to get an STD.

Most people don't realize how easy it is to get an STD until they get one themselves. Your chances of becoming infected by an STD are increased if you have sexual contact with:

- Someone you have just met or hardly know.
- Someone with whom you have not discussed your concerns about STDs.
- Someone who has had many partners over a short period of time.
- Someone who appears to have STD symptoms.
- Many partners over a short period of time.

## How can I reduce my risk of getting an STD?

Getting to know your partner before having sexual contact will reduce your risk of getting an STD.

Whenever possible, do not engage in sexual activity with someone until you have gotten to know him or her over a period of a month or more. Also, try to find out if your potential partner has been sexually involved with anyone else during that period. If your partner has an STD from a previous sexual contact, it may become noticeable during the first few weeks of your relationship, and thus could be treated before you risk getting it yourself.

As you get to know your partner, you will get a better sense of his or her sexual values and behavior. For example, while you may limit the number of your sexual contacts, your partner may not do the same. Once you know what sort of risks are involved in relating to a potential partner, you can decide whether you want to begin (or continue) to have a sexual relationship with this person.

Try to talk openly about disease prevention before engaging in close contact with someone you hardly know. Discuss your beliefs and feelings with your prospective partner. Ask if he or she has ever had an STD. Find out what sort of knowledge the person has about STDs. And, to play it safe, use a condom whenever you have sexual contact with someone who is not your exclusive partner.

Of course, not having sexual contact with anyone is always an option.

## Is there a vaccine to prevent STDs?

At present, there is no vaccine to prevent any form of STD except hepatitis B. (The hepatitis B vaccine became available in 1982 after extensive testing.)

Researchers are hopeful that vaccines will be developed for gonorrhea and herpes within the next few years.

**Can I take antibiotics or other medicine to prevent STDs?**

There is no medicine that you can take to prevent STDs.

Taking antibiotics to prevent STDs is risky for several reasons:

- Each disease is different, and requires a different type of antibiotic to treat.
- Proper dosages vary from one person to another and, especially, from one disease to another.
- The overuse of antibiotics can actually make some infections more difficult to cure because organisms may become resistant to the drug's effect.
- Some people who take large quantities of antibiotics develop allergies or sensitivities to these drugs, which can result in life-threatening reactions.
- Antibiotics may kill organisms that are beneficial to you, such as certain bacteria in the intestines.

**How can I protect myself from STDs during sexual activity?**

Although there is no guaranteed way to prevent STDs, the following measures will reduce your chances of getting an infection:

- Wash before and immediately after sexual contact. Pay special attention to your hands and genitals, and wash out your mouth after oral sex. Washing helps remove surface bacteria that may be present.
- Urinate after sexual contact. This is often helpful in preventing STDs in men, since it washes bacteria from the urinary opening. This technique is less effective in women, due to differences in female anatomy.
- Use a condom. Condoms can help protect both men and women from some, but not all, STDs. Many women now keep condoms in their purse to make sure that they have one available if needed.

**Am I more likely to get an STD when I have another illness?**

Most diseases lower your resistance to infection. Therefore, if you are ill, even with a common cold or flu, you should be extra careful to avoid exposure to STDs.

**Can fatigue and stress cause STDs?**

No. Fatigue and stress do not, by themselves, cause STDs, but they can dramatically reduce your resistance to infections in general. To get an infection you must be exposed to a virus, bacteria, or other disease-causing agent.

Fatigue and stress are known to affect herpes in particular. People who have herpes are more likely to have outbreaks when they are feeling tired or under pressure.

Reducing stress through rest and relaxation is important in maintaining your resistance to disease.

**Are drug and alcohol use related to getting STDs?**

Drugs and alcohol do not cause STDs, but they do lower your resistance to disease in general.

In addition, if you are under the influence of drugs and/or alcohol, you may not be able to exercise your best judgment concerning whether or not to engage in sexual activity. Even worse, you might become infected during a sexual experience that you have forgotten by the next morning.

**Will vitamins and minerals protect me from STDs?**

Vitamins and minerals can contribute to your overall good health, thus helping to build your resistance to disease. However, there are no known vitamins or minerals, or combinations of the two, that can prevent STDs.

Some people who suffer from recurrent herpes believe that vitamins and minerals help prevent flare-ups of the disease. This may be true, since flare-ups seem to be related to stress, and vitamin/mineral supplements appear to help reduce stress.

Keep in mind that poor nutrition is a form of bodily stress that may increase your risk of becoming infected. While a well-balanced diet is your best defense against poor nutrition, dietary supplements may also be helpful. If you decide you want to take vitamin/mineral supplements, it is advisable to see a health professional to determine which ones will best meet your needs.

**Can wearing certain kinds of clothes affect my risk of getting STDs?**

Yes. Tight-fitting clothes worn around the genital area can increase your risk of infection.

The health of the genitals is dependent upon maintaining certain temperature and moisture levels in the genital area. Wearing tight underclothes, nylon pantyhose, and tight polyester pants raises the temperature and moisture level around the genitals, thus lowering your resistance to disease. A hot, moist environment also encourages the growth of yeast, bacteria, and viruses.

Loose clothing and soft, cotton underwear are not only comfortable, but help to prevent bacterial and viral infection. Of course no form of clothing can prevent you from getting infections that are transmitted by direct contact with someone who has an STD.

**Can douches prevent STDs?**

No. Douches do not prevent STDs.

Doctors sometimes prescribe douches to treat conditions in which there is an imbalance of organisms that normally live in the vagina, but these douches do not provide protection against STDs. In fact, the misuse of douches can force vaginal organisms into the cervix (the muscular opening to the uterus), further complicating an already existing infection.

Perfumed douches may be particularly risky. These do nothing to prevent infection, and have been known to irritate sensitive vaginal tissue.

**Can contraceptive jellies, creams, and foams prevent STDs?**

While these contraceptives act as barriers against sperm and/or kill sperm in order to prevent pregnancy, none of them can be relied upon to prevent STDs.

**Can birth control pills prevent STDs?**

No. Birth control pills are a form of contraception. When used properly, they help prevent pregnancy, nothing more.

## Will a diaphragm help prevent STDs?

A diaphragm may *temporarily* prevent the spread of infection, but as soon as it is removed, any organisms that have entered the vaginal canal can easily spread to the cervix and to other parts of the body.

**Can an IUD help prevent STDs?**

No. An IUD is intended only to prevent pregnancy, not disease.

It is important to be aware that IUD use increases the risk of pelvic infection in women by providing a means of entry for bacteria and other organisms that move along the IUD "string" that leads through the cervix to the inside of the uterus. If a woman who uses an IUD has numerous sexual partners, the risk of infection is even greater. For this reason, IUDs are recommended primarily for women who have only one, long-term sexual partner.

If you are considering using an IUD, it is important to discuss the advantages and disadvantages of this form of contraception with a medical professional. Try to be honest and open about your sexual activity so that you can get a realistic idea of the potential risks involved in IUD use.

**Can condoms help prevent STDs?**

The condom is the best available means of preventing STDs.

Anything that minimizes direct genital contact during sexual activity reduces the risk of getting STDs. While condoms do not provide 100% protection, when used according to the instructions provided, they are the best protection available.

The condom provides a physical barrier between the man's penis and his partner. If either partner is infected in areas that do not come in contact with the condom, infection can, of course, still be spread from one person to another.

Condoms are most effective against chlamydia, gonorrhea, nongonococcal urethritis, and trichomoniasis, and can provide limited protection against hepatitis B, herpes, syphilis, and venereal warts. Condoms will not protect you from scabies, crabs, or other diseases not restricted to the genital area.

**What are the advantages of using condoms?**

Condoms are easy to buy and easy to use.

- They are readily available. You can buy condoms from display racks in drug stores and supermarkets and by mail order.
- They can be conveniently carried in pocket, purse, or wallet. (Be careful that the packet does not accidentally break open and expose or puncture the condom!)
- They are easy to put on; instructions are provided with the condom box.
- They provide an effective barrier against some STDs (and also help to prevent pregnancy).
- They have no side effects; some people are allergic to lubricated or dyed condoms, but in these cases, nonlubricated or "plain" condoms can be used.

# CHAPTER FOUR

# JUST THE TWO OF YOU

## How do I find out if my new partner has an STD?

Open communication is the best way to find out if your partner may have an STD.

Before entering into a relationship that will include sexual intimacy, discuss the subject of STDs with your new partner. Find out what your partner knows about STDs. Has he or she ever had an STD in the past? Does he or she undergo routine testing for STDs by a health professional? Consider your partner's responses to these questions and compare them to your own experience. You can save yourself a lot of future problems by deciding not to engage in sexual activity until you have established a good understanding with your new partner.

Be alert to outward signs and symptoms that might lead you to suspect that a potential partner may be an STD carrier. To be absolutely safe, you and your partner may want to visit a health professional together at the start of your relationship to be sure that you are both in good health and present no threat of infection to each other.

**How can I begin a conversation about STDs with my partner?**

Sometimes it is not easy to start this kind of conversation. If you are uncomfortable about it, try to ease into the subject by asking questions such as:

"Have you seen all of the newspaper stories about herpes lately?"

"Have you ever had herpes or anything like that?"

"Do you have any diseases I should know about?"

"Do you have sexual relations very often?"

"Do you ever worry about getting a sexually transmitted disease?"

Make it clear that you are concerned about your partner's health as well as your own.

**What STD symptoms should I look for in a partner?**

Symptoms in the genital area that should cause you to ask further questions or decline sexual contact include:

- Complaints of discomfort
- A sore, rash, or discharge
- Unusual odors
- Swelling and/or redness

**Can someone with no STD symptoms still be contagious?**

Yes. The absence of symptoms does not mean that a person is not contagious.

For example, most women who have chlamydia or gonorrhea do not know they are infected, but can still pass on their infection to another person.

With some diseases—herpes, for example—there may be a period of time just prior to an outbreak of symptoms when the infected person is contagious. Usually, but not always, an outbreak will be preceded by warning signs such as tingling or burning in the genital area.

**Can I get an STD from someone who claims not to have one?**

Yes. Not everyone who has an STD knows it.

Many infected people honestly believe they are uninfected because they have no noticeable symptoms. The absence of symptoms, however, is no guarantee of the absence of disease. Also, of course, some people may know that they have an infection, but choose not to tell you about it.

**When is it safe to have sexual contact with someone who has an STD?**

An infected person remains contagious until the STD is completely cured.

Sexual contact is not safe until the infected person has undergone medical testing and has been given a "clean bill of health" by a health professional. Just because someone is taking medication does not mean that the infection is gone.

In general, both partners (and anyone else who has had intimate contact with the infected person) should be tested, and treated if necessary. Because symptoms do not always show up immediately, the partner who appears to be uninfected may later prove to have the infection, and thus unknowingly pass it back to the originally infected partner. This cycle could go on indefinitely.

If your partner has ever had herpes, he or she may have periodic outbreaks of the disease. You should not have any sexual contact during the contagious period, which includes several days *before* a flare-up, as well as the outbreak itself.

**Is penetration or orgasm necessary to get an STD?**

While penetration means added intimate contact, it is not necessary in order to pass on an STD. Any form of physical intimacy or skin-to-skin contact can transmit an STD from one person to another.

Having an orgasm is not necessary to spread the infection.

**Can couples who are not having sexual contact with other people get STDs?**

Yes. It is possible for a couple to become infected even if no other sexual contacts are involved.

If one partner has had an STD in the past (knowingly or unknowingly), the disease may recur at some time in the future. (Herpes and venereal warts, for example, can both recur over time.) If neither person has ever been infected, there is very little chance of disease. Should an infection occur (or recur), open conversation, trust, and understanding are very important.

Crabs and scabies can both be passed on through nonsexual contact, and therefore should not be regarded as evidence that a partner has had sexual relations with someone else.

Other diseases that affect the genital area but are not necessarily sexually transmitted include bladder infections, candidiasis in women, and prostatitis in men.

## Can I get STDs from anal or oral sex?

Yes. STDs can be spread through both anal and oral sex.

Disease-causing organisms can be found in the mouth, in the anus, and on the genitals, and can be passed on to another person. For example, oral herpes can be transmitted to the genitals in oral-genital sex.

Many infections are transmitted by waste matter and by blood. Because some bleeding is often associated with anal sex, infecting organisms have relatively easy entry into the body and may well lead to the spread of infection. As a result, there is a relatively high risk of spreading STDs through anal-genital sex. Infections can also be transmitted from the anus to the mouth, and vice versa.

Because waste matter may be contaminated with blood and disease-causing organisms, partners who engage in anal or oral sex should thoroughly wash their mouths and genital and anal areas immediately following this type of sexual activity to prevent the spread of infection.

**Do most people try to protect their partners from getting STDs?**

In general, people do not intentionally spread STDs to their partners.

Although STDs may trigger all sorts of emotions, particularly fear and embarrassment, most people will take the necessary steps to protect their partners. This may mean the consistent use of condoms; it may mean avoiding sexual activity; or it may mean you and your partner visiting a physician or clinic for checkups.

Because of the increasing number of cases and growing seriousness of STDs, anyone who is sexually active should talk to their partner about potential problems related to these diseases. It is especially important to talk about how you and your partner can protect each other from getting and spreading STDs.

Sometimes a person will not want to tell his or her partner about an infection that is diagnosed after the two have engaged in sexual activity. If you are in this situation, one way to deal with it is to give your partner's name and address to your local health department, and ask that they notify him or her. This valuable service, provided by a public health specialist, can often break the chain of infection by informing the sexual partners of infected people.

## CHAPTER FIVE

# IF YOU THINK YOU HAVE AN STD . . .

**How can I tell if I have an STD?**

If you know the symptoms associated with STDs, you will know when to suspect a possible infection.

Many symptoms that are associated with STDs can also be caused by other diseases that are not related to sexual activity. The only way to know for sure if you have an STD is to have a medical examination. (Don't wait and "hope it will go away.") The following symptoms may be caused by an STD and should be checked by a health professional:

- Burning or pain in the genitals, anus, or rectum
- Pain in the abdomen during sexual activity
- Unusual discharge from the vagina or penis
- Sores, growths, warts, rashes, or itching in the mouth or in the anal or genital areas

The following symptoms are probably *not* indications of STDs but should be checked by a health professional if there is reason to suspect that you might have an STD or any other disease:

- Sores, growths, warts, rashes, or itching on any part of the body other than in the mouth or in the anal or genital areas
- Flu-like symptoms including aching, pain in the joints, diarrhea, fever

**How long does it take for symptoms to appear after I am exposed to an STD?**

Many symptoms are noticed within a week after exposure; however, it can take as long as one month or more for some symptoms to appear. The length of time between exposure and appearance of symptoms varies from disease to disease and from person to person.

**If I have pain during sexual activity, do I have an STD?**

Pain is not necessarily a symptom of STDs, but it can be. In any case, pain that is experienced during sexual activity is not normal, and should be discussed with a health professional.

**If I have pain when urinating, do I have an STD?**

Pain during urination is a very common symptom of STDs in men. However, this symptom also can be caused by other conditions, such as bladder infections. Any discomfort when urinating should be checked by a health professional.

**If my partner gets an STD, will I get it too?**

If you have sexual contact with someone who has an STD, there is a good chance that you will get it, too. For this reason, both you and your partner should have a medical check-up at the same time.

## What should I do if I think I have an STD?

First of all, stop all sexual activity, and second, get prompt medical attention at a clinic, doctor's office, or neighborhood health center.

If you do not seek immediate treatment, the more obvious symptoms of your condition may disappear, making a diagnosis more difficult. Also, the longer you wait to be examined, the more likely it is that your condition will become more serious, and therefore more difficult to treat. It is important to remember that you may be infected even if you have no noticeable symptoms.

If you are being treated for an STD, be sure to follow medical instructions carefully. Take all medication you are given, for as long as you are directed to do so. Do not use old medication or share your medication with anyone else.

When seeking medical treatment, there is no need to be concerned about giving personal information to a physician or health professional, since these people are required by law to keep the names of their patients confidential.

If you are upset or distressed about having an STD, you may want to talk to a trained counselor. Your local VD clinic may offer counseling services; if not, they can tell you whom to contact.

**If I do get an STD, can it be cured?**

Most STDs are easily cured with the proper antibiotic therapy.

Diseases that are caused by a virus, such as hepatitis B, herpes, and AIDS, cannot yet be cured. Researchers are still attempting to develop medications that will effectively treat these diseases.

**How can I help prevent the spread of infection to others if I know I have an STD?**

As soon as you know you are infected, you must take immediate steps to prevent the further spread of disease.

Contact your sexual partner(s) of the past month (or whatever time period your doctor says you may have been contagious) and let them know that you may have spread the infection to them. This is the only way to ensure that your sexual contacts are treated as soon as possible.

Make sure that you receive proper medical treatment, and return for check-ups as directed. Never assume that you are cured until your health professional says that you are.

Do not resume sexual activity until a follow-up examination indicates that your disease has been cured.

**If I ignore STD symptoms, will they go away?**

Symptoms may disappear temporarily, but the infection will not go away unless it is treated.

Symptoms can reappear weeks or months later if the disease is still present. The disappearance of symptoms does not mean that an infection is gone; it may be present in your bloodstream or in other parts of your body.

If symptoms are ignored, complications may develop later, making the disease more difficult to treat. If an infection goes untreated, it can result in serious, irreversible damage, the most common being sterility in both men and women; some untreated STD cases may even result in death.

## What do people think about someone who gets an STD?

There are as many different thoughts about getting STDs as there are people.

Some people believe that getting an STD is "proper punishment" for what they consider to be improper, immoral, or deviant behavior. Other people feel that someone who is infected has been deliberately victimized. Because STDs are passed on through sexual contact, they are frequently viewed with a mixture of embarrassment, fear, ignorance, and moral judgment.

People who understand the principles of sexually transmitted disease generally believe that, in most cases, STDs are simply passed on by an unsuspecting partner.

## STDs AT A GLANCE

A brief description of these diseases can be found in the *Definitions of Terms and Diseases* section, which follows.

| Name of Disease | Effectively Treatable if Diagnosed Early? | Curable in 1 to 4 weeks? |
|---|---|---|
| AIDS | no | no |
| *Candidiasis (Monilia or yeast) | yes | yes |
| Chancroid | yes | yes |
| *Chlamydia | yes | yes |
| *Crabs | yes | yes |
| Cytomegalovirus | no | goes away but may recur |
| Epstein-Barr Virus | no | goes away but may recur |
| *Gardnerella vaginalis | yes | yes |
| *Gonorrhea | yes | yes |
| Granuloma inguinale | yes | yes |

*most common STDs

| Name of Disease | Effectively Treatable if Diagnosed Early? | Curable in 1 to 4 weeks? |
|---|---|---|
| *Herpes (genital or labial) | yes | goes away but may recur |
| Lymphogranuloma Venereum (LGV) | yes | yes |
| Molluscum contagiosum | yes | yes |
| *Nongonococcal Urethritis (NGU) | yes | yes |
| *Pelvic Inflammatory Disease (PID) | yes | yes |
| Scabies | yes | yes |
| *Syphilis | yes | yes |
| *Trichomoniasis | yes | yes |
| *Vaginitis | yes | yes |
| *Venereal Warts | yes | goes away but may recur |
| *Viral Hepatitis | yes | not Hepatitis B |

*most common STDs

## WHERE TO GET MORE HELP

**1. Health professionals (medical advice and treatment)**

Clinics

Listed in Telephone Book (yellow pages)—see *Clinics, Health Clinics, Hospitals,* or go to your local Teen Clinic or the student health center at your college.

Planned Parenthood

Listed in Telephone Book (white pages)—see *Planned Parenthood*.

Private Physicians

Listed in Telephone Book (yellow pages)—call your doctor or see *Physicians and Surgeons* listings; or call your *County Medical Society* (for a referral).

Public Health Department

Listed in Telephone Book (white pages)—see City, County, or State listings: *Health Department, Public Health Department, Venereal Disease.*

**2. General Information about STDs**

VD National Hotline

—In California (800) 982-5883

—Rest of United States 1 (800) 227-8922

**3. Information about AIDS**

AIDS Hotline

—In New York (212) 807-6016

—Rest of United States 1 (800) 221-7044

**4. Books about STDs**

Local Bookstore—*Health* Section

Local public library or school library—
See *Venereal Disease* in card catalog.

**5. Psychological Counseling**

Private psychiatrists and psychologists
Listed in Telephone Book (yellow pages)—see *Physicians and Surgeons* listings: *Psychiatrists* or *County Medical Society* (for a referral), or see *Psychologists*.

Social Services
Listed in Telephone Book (white pages)—See City, County or State listings: *Mental Health, Social Services*.

**6. Crisis Help**

Crisis Hotlines or Crisis Intervention Centers
Listed in Telephone Book (yellow pages)—see *Crisis Hotline* or call Directory Assistance (411).

## DEFINITIONS OF TERMS AND DISEASES

The following definitions are provided to give you a general understanding of commonly used terminology related to sexually transmitted diseases. These definitions are not intended to serve as comprehensive medical explanations, and not all terms are used in the text.

**AIDS (Acquired Immunodeficiency Syndrome):** A disease which is often sexually transmitted and results in the breakdown of the body's normal defense mechanisms against infection (the immune system). Certain tumors are sometimes associated with this disease, as are numerous other serious medical problems.

**Antibiotic:** An agent made from mold or bacteria that destroys or slows the growth of bacteria. Antibiotics are used as medication to fight bacterial infections such as gonorrhea and syphilis, but are not effective in treating viral infections.

**Anus:** The lower opening of the digestive tract through which waste matter passes.

**Asymptomatic:** Showing no symptoms of disease. This word is often used to describe infections that produce no noticeable symptoms.

**Autoinnoculation:** Reinfection of oneself by spreading organisms from one part of the body to another.

**Bacterium (plural, bacteria):** Microscopic organisms, or microorganisms. Some microorganisms cause infection in humans, and some help fight or prevent infection or are beneficial in other ways.

**Bladder:** The organ that holds urine until it is passed from the body.

**Candidiasis (monilia or yeast):** A fungal infection of the skin and mucous membranes.

**Causative agent:** As used in this book, a causative agent is any virus, bacteria, or other organism that produces disease (for example, the gonococcus bacterium causes gonorrhea). A causative agent is also referred to as a *pathogen*.

**Cervix:** The lower, neck-like, muscular portion of the uterus, connecting it with the vagina.

**Chancre (pronounced "shanker"):** A sore, usually painless, that forms in the area at which spirochetes (microorganisms that cause syphilis) enter the body; also referred to as *hard chancre*, to distinguish it from the *soft chancre* of chancroid.

**Chancroid:** A bacterial STD that causes a painful, pus-filled bump, sometimes referred to as a *soft chancre*.

**Chlamydia:** An organism that causes a series of diseases that result in the development of painful enlargements of the lymph nodes and other symptoms. The STDs lymphogranuloma venereum (LGV) and nongonococcal urethritis (NGU) are caused by chlamydia.

**Coitus:** See *Intercourse, sexual*.

**Communicable:** Capable of being passed from one person to another.

**Condom:** A thin rubber sheath that covers the erect penis during sexual activity to help protect against infection and/or pregnancy. Sometimes referred to as a *rubber* or *prophylactic*.

**Congenital:** Present at birth.

**Contact:** As used in this book, contact refers to anyone with whom an infected person has had sexual intercourse or other close physical contact.

**Culture:** As used in this book, culture refers to a process of medical testing during which organisms taken from an infected person's body are grown in a laboratory in order to identify them.

**Cytomegalovirus:** A type of herpes virus.

**Diagnosis:** Medical identification of a disease, syndrome, or condition based on descriptions of symptoms, physical examination, and observation of signs, laboratory tests, and/or an interview with the patient.

**Douche:** Cleansing of the vagina with liquid—usually water—that is sometimes medicated. Commercial preparations may contain perfume and other additives that can be irritating to the soft, moist tissue of the vagina.

**Ejaculation:** The discharge of semen from the penis during orgasm.

**Epidemic:** The spread of a disease to many people in a community simultaneously.

**Epstein-Barr virus:** A type of herpes virus. Epstein-Barr herpetovirus may cause mononucleosis.

**Fallopian tubes:** Tubes leading from the ovaries to the uterus, along which the egg (ovum) travels.

**Gardnerella vaginalis:** A highly contagious, but not serious vaginal bacterial infection that causes a discharge and irritation.

**Gay:** See *Homosexual.*

**Genital herpes:** An infection, caused by the herpes simplex virus, that affects the genitals.

**Genitals:** The reproductive organs; sex organs.

**Gonococcus:** The bacterium that causes gonorrhea.

**Gonorrhea:** A serious STD that affects both men and women, causing swelling of the urethral lining, the vagina and other genital organs in women, and sometimes the mouth and rectum; it is caused by the gonococcus bacterium.

**Granuloma inguinale:** A bacterial STD that causes inflamed sores in the genital and perianal region.

**Hemophilia:** A congenital (present at birth) blood disorder in which the blood is unable to form clots. A person who has hemophilia (a hemophiliac, or "bleeder") may lose a substantial amount of blood from a small wound.

**Hepatitis B:** See *Viral hepatitis.*

**Herpes simplex virus:** A virus that causes localized infection in the form of a painful sore on the lips or genitals. The infection may recur periodically over an individual's lifetime.

**Homosexual:** A person who prefers to have sexual relations with others of the same sex; relating to sexual relations with a person of the same sex. Also referred to as *Gay.*

**Immunity:** Ability of the body to resist infection.

**Incubation period:** The time it takes for disease symptoms to appear following infection by a virus, bacterium, or other disease-causing agent.

**Infectious:** Contagious; able to spread from one person to another; used to describe diseases.

**Intercourse, sexual:** Physical activity involving sexual arousal and contact between the genitals of two people of the opposite sex in which the penis is inserted into the vagina.

**Intrauterine device (IUD):** A device inserted in the uterus and left there to prevent conception.

**Labial herpes:** Localized infection around the mouth and lips caused by herpes simplex virus.

**Lesion:** A sore, wound, or injury.

**Lymphogranuloma venereum (LGV):** STD caused by the organism *Chlamydia trachomatis*.

**Molluscum contagiosum:** An infectious disease that causes small, hard bumps under the skin.

**Mucous membrane:** A layer of soft, moist skin inside the mouth, nose, vagina, and anus, as well as in other parts of the body.

**Neonatal infection:** Infection of newborns. If the mother is infected at the time of delivery, the infection may spread to the baby as it passes through the birth canal.

**Nongonococcal urethritis (NGU):** Infections of the urethra caused by microorganisms other than the gonococcus bacterium (which causes gonorrhea); often caused by chlamydia.

**Orgasm:** The peak or climax of sexual excitement, experienced by both sexes. Rhythmic, muscular contractions occur, and the sensation is intensely pleasurable. A man usually ejaculates during orgasm.

**Ovaries:** Female sex glands that produce egg cells (ova) and certain hormones.

**Ovum (plural, ova):** An egg cell.

**Parasite:** An organism that lives on or in another organism (the host), and usually is dependent on the host for survival. Parasites are often, but not always, detrimental to the host's well being.

**Pelvic inflammatory disease (PID):** Inflammation of the pelvic organs in women that may cause scarring and may result in sterility. Sometimes affects the fallopian tubes.

**Penis:** Male sex organ.

**Promiscuous:** Having sex with several partners within a short period of time. Often means indiscriminate choice of partners.

**Prostitute:** A person who is paid for performing sexual acts, including intercourse.

**Rectum:** The lower end of the digestive tract, between the large intestine (colon) and the anus.

**Salpingitis:** Inflammation of the fallopian tubes.

**Scabies:** Skin eruptions, irritation, and itching caused by mites—tiny insects that burrow into the skin.

**Semen (seminal fluid):** Pale, milk-colored fluid that contains sperm cells and is ejaculated by the male during orgasm.

**Sex, anal-genital:** Insertion of the penis through the anus into the rectum of another person.

**Sex, oral-anal:** Sexual contact between the mouth and tongue of one person and the anus of another person.

**Sex, oral-genital:** Sexual contact between the mouth and tongue of one person and the genitals of another person.

**Sexual contact:** Intimate contact between two people involving sexual arousal and any form of sexual activity.

**Sexual intercourse:** See *Intercourse, sexual.*

**Spirochete:** A bacterium that causes syphilis.

**Syphilis:** A serious bacterial STD. If untreated, the disease spreads throughout the body and affects many organs, including the brain; can be fatal.

**Trichomoniasis (Trich):** A disease caused by the organism *Trichomonas*, which infects the vagina and/or urethra. Usually causes a discharge, and can affect both men and women.

**Uterus (womb):** The part of the female reproductive system in which a baby develops.

**Vaccine:** A medical preparation that contains weakened or killed organisms, such as viruses. When a vaccine enters the body, it stimulates the immune system to form *antibodies*, which protect the body against invasion by the particular organism used.

**Vagina:** The passage leading from outside the woman's body to the uterus.

**Vaginitis:** Any inflammation of the vagina; may or may not be caused by an STD.

**VDRL (Venereal Disease Research Laboratories) test:** A test for syphilis.

**Venereal:** Related to the sex organs (from the Latin, *Venus*, the goddess of love).

**Venereal disease (VD):** Another term for sexually transmitted disease (STD).

**Venereal warts:** Cauliflower-shaped warts in the genital area; a highly contagious viral STD.

**Viral hepatitis:** A viral infection that results in inflammation of the liver. It can be transmitted through blood or bodily fluids. Hepatitis B is one form of viral hepatitis.

**Virus:** An infectious agent that relies on normal body cells to grow and reproduce.

# INDEX

# THE AUTHORS

## Bea Mandel, R.N., M.P.H.

In August 1979, Bea Mandel established a national VD Hotline based in Palo Alto, California. Supported in part by a federal grant from the Centers for Disease Control and the American Social Health Association (a United Way Agency), the Hotline became a national, all-volunteer program created to answer questions about sexually transmitted diseases.

As director of the VD National Hotline for over four years, Bea developed STD training programs for people from all walks of life to help them provide information and referral services to callers from all over the country.

Prior to establishing the Hotline, Bea was a faculty member in the Health Sciences Department at San Jose State University, where she specialized in Community Health Education. She is presently the Director of the Department of Education at the Seton Medical Center in Daly City, California, where she is responsible for educational programs at the Medical Center and within the community-at-large.

## Byron Mandel

Byron Mandel has been a volunteer supervisor for the VD National Hotline in Palo Alto, California, where he has provided counseling and referrals to thousands of callers seeking information about sexually transmitted diseases.

The Mandels are not related.

## THE AUTHORS

[illegible]

[illegible] Mexican [illegible] National [illegible]

[illegible] the country.

Prior to [illegible] member of the [illegible] Medical Center [illegible] Department of [illegible] responsible for [illegible] programs at the Mexican [illegible]

[illegible]

[illegible] Alto, California. [illegible] knowledge of [illegible] information about Central American [illegible]

[illegible] made [illegible] possible.

## REMEMBER . . .

**STDs are highly contagious.**

**The risk of getting STDs is greater than ever.**

**Be alert to STD symptoms on your own body and on your partner's body.**

**Use caution when considering a new sexual partner.**

**Protect yourself from STDs before, during, and after sexual activity.**

**Get medical attention as soon as you suspect that you have an infection.**

**Notify your recent sexual partners if you find that you do have an infection.**

**Get a checkup for STDs twice a year— more often if you are sexually active and have multiple partners.**

## MAY WE HAVE YOUR COMMENTS?

We would very much appreciate receiving any comments you may have about *Play Safe*. Your comments will help make future editions of this book more valuable to our readers.

- Did you enjoy reading the book?
- Did you find the book informative?
- Has this information been useful?

If there is any additional information you would like to see included in our next, updated edition, please let us know. Unfortunately, we cannot answer questions by phone or mail. If you need immediate assistance, we recommend that you contact one of the resources listed in "Where to Get More Help" at the back of this book.

If you would like to provide us with your name and address, we would be happy to put you on our mailing list and notify you about our future publications.

Play safe, and be well.

Center for Health Information
P.O. Box 4636
Foster City, CA 94404